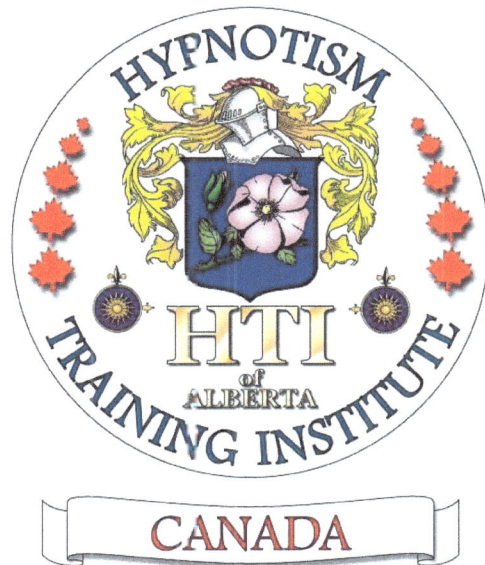

Hypnosis 201

Professional
Hypnotism

By Anny J. Slegten

Professional Hypnotism
Anny Slegten
Published by
Kimberlite Publishing House
www.kimberlitePublishingHouse.com

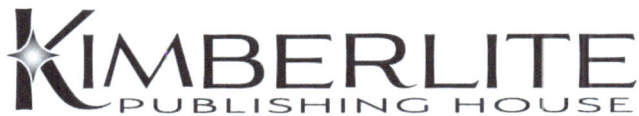

KIMBERLITE
PUBLISHING HOUSE

ISBN: 978-1-7752489-5-8

School Coat of Arms designed by Boomer Stralak
Book layout by Colin Christopher *www.colinchristopher.com*
Book cover and Kimberlite Logo designed by Marietta Miller
www.execugraphx.com

The Kimberlite-Diamond Connection

Kimberlite is a rock type that was first categorized over a 100 years ago based on descriptions of the diamond-bearing pipes of Kimberley, South Africa.

Kimberlites are the mechanism by which diamonds are brought to the surface.

Kimberlitic rocks are the most important primary source of diamonds and the main rock type in which significant diamond deposits have been found so far.

Anny is familiar with many rocks and minerals as her husband was raised around quarries, and later worked in several mines in Canada.

Therefore, it was natural for Anny to choose kimberlite as an analogy to the soul residing within our body – as a diamond within the kimberlite.

A Picture Is Worth A Thousand Words

Seeing the Buddha facing the front of my office, surrounded by bright yellow Marigolds, someone asked me if I was a Buddhist.

No, I am not a Buddhist was my answer.

Well said the visitor who came at the door to sell me recently taken aerial pictures of the property, how come then do you have a Buddha there?

I chose to put this friendly and smiling Buddha there to convey my welcome to friends, clients, and student.

The peace of Buddha is the perfect welcome onto the fascinating and rewarding world of hypnosis.

As you are holding this book in your hands, I welcome you to the next step in your hypnosis journey!

Anny

Welcome to

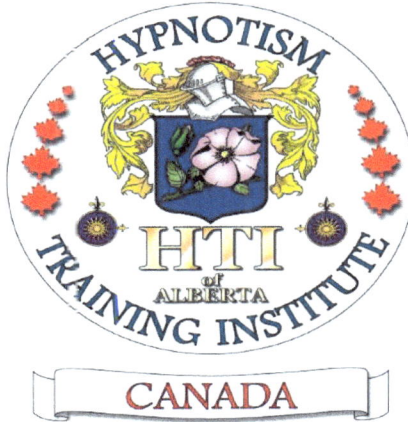

HYP 201 – Professional Hypnotism

This book belongs to:

Name _____

Mailing Address _____

_____

City or Town _____

Province/State _____ Postal Code/Zip _____

Country _____

Telephone Home (___) _____ Work (___) _____

Instructor's Name: ***Anny Slegten***

Today's Date: _____

Table Of Contents

A Note From Anny

The design and development of the Course Material required the investment of substantial effort, time and money and is only intended for the participants of HYP 201, Professional Hypnotism.

Understand that the experiences derived from attending this course is a private and personal experience for each participant. As such please do respect the confidentiality of all participants and their remarks and actions and keep all such information private and confidential.

As a result, I am counting on you do your part at keeping this course environment safe and secure for all participants.

Enjoy!

Empty Your Cup

A professor from a University went to visit a famous Zen master.

While the master quietly served tea, the professor talked about Zen.

The master poured the visitor's cup to the brim and then kept pouring.

The professor watched the overflowing cup until he could no longer restrain himself.

'It is overfull! No more will go in!' the professor blurted.

'You are like this cup,' the Master replied, 'How can I show you Zen unless you first empty your cup.'

Your Notes

Anny's Teaching

Confidentiality

I, the undersigned, understand that the experiences derived from attending this course is a private and personal experience for each participant. I hereby promise to respect the confidentiality of all participants, their remarks and their actions and keep all such information private and confidential. As a result, I promise to do my part at keeping this course environment safe and secure for all participants.

I intend this commitment to apply to all my present and future Hypnotism and Reiki classes.

Name _____ Date of Birth _____

Mailing address _____

City/Town _____

Province _____

Postal Code _____

Telephone (Home) _____

(Work) _____

(Cellular) _____

Occupation _____

E-mail address _____

_____   _____
Signature   Today's Date

Your Notes

Anny's Teaching

Hypnotism and Reiki Seminars & Certification Programs
Release and Consent Form

Hypnosis, self-hypnosis, regression, past life regression, guided visualization, and clinical depossession are clinical modalities, and when used appropriately have been known to benefit people. These and other techniques may be used in this workshop, with the highest integrity and appropriateness. If you do have any problems or upsets during this workshop, please notify the instructor. It is our intention that this workshop be a beneficial learning and healing experience for all participants.

_____

I, the undersigned, understand that lectures, demonstrations and experiential processes may stimulate personal issues.

I take full responsibility for any treatment that I may wish to engage in as a result of recognizing these issues.

I understand that this seminar may be videotaped and/or audiotaped. I hereby grant permission to Anny Slegten to use any part of this video or audio tape which might include me, for any videotape, cassette tape, film, article, book, or lecture on the subject of hypnosis, self-hypnosis, regression, past life regression, guided visualization, and clinical depossession. I understand they may be sold for a profit. I reserve the right to have my name removed from the tape providing I give advance written notice to that effect. I promise to hold harmless Anny Slegten, The Seminar and Retreat Organizers, The Reiki Training Centre of Canada, the Hypnotism Training Institute of Alberta (1989), Success ... & More Hypnotherapy and Motivation Clinic, any participants or assistants at this seminar, for any problems that may occur or stemming from this seminar.

I intend this waiver to apply to all my present and future Reiki and Hypnosis/Hypnotherapy seminars.

Name (please print) _____

Address _____

City _____ Province _____

Postal Code _____ Occupation _____

Telephone Home _____ Work _____

Facsimile _____ E-mail _____

Date _____ Signature _____

Your Notes

Anny's Teaching

Hypnosis Vs. Hypnotherapy Part 1
What is the difference?

By Anny Slegten, Master Hypnotist, Clinical Hypnotherapist

Public awareness of hypnosis has greatly improved since I opened my hypnosis and hypnotherapy practice in 1984.

At the time, the moment I mentioned I was a hypnotherapist, people would cover their eyes, turn their head and say 'Don't look at me!'

I would just answer, 'Relax. I charge!' This reminds me of a cartoon one of my students gave me: a couple is having a drink on the terrace of a café. Starry eyes, the lady says to the gentleman, 'Are you trying to tell me you can make me come by just gazing into my i-yi-yi-yi-yieees?.

Wow! Would it be nice to have power like that: just look at them in the eyes and make them do whatever people think I can make them do. Who wants to be accountable when there is no success? You, like me, believe in freedom of choice, whatever the choice may be.

What is hypnosis? Hypnosis is consciously going into an altered sate of awareness, a trance. It can be used as a tool, as a technique, or both. Hypnosis in its versability can be used in many ways, and for this article, let us consider hypnosis as a technique.

By relaxing the conscious mind, we can consciously plant a suggestion into our subconscious mind. Once you are aware of that ability, you can have terrific conversations with the different parts of yourself. This can be highly entertaining!

Your Notes

Anny's Teaching

Having emotionalised thoughts is a powerful way to plant suggestions, and staying conscious in the moment allows us to program ourselves with what we want.

Presenting suggestions so the conscious mind will accept them is an art and is not as easy to do as one is made to believe, for to go subconscious it must have the co-operation of the conscious mind who is acting as the 'sensor, or the 'gate keeper'.

It is possible to be in a deep trance and not follow suggestions. Therefore, no matter how. deep the trance, there must be co-operation. Yes, you are always in control, whether you like it or not So I ask you, how come people make such fools of themselves with stage hypnosis? I can be wide-awake and do that all by myself! How about you?

Hypnosis is always self-hypnosis: The only one who can hypnotise you is you.

Hypnosis removes inhibitions and that is how it is so valuable in many situations. For example, going into hypnosis just before public speaking helps in the delivery of the presentation. This process is sometimes called "Self-psyching".

Using self-hypnosis for relaxation allows the body to regulate itself, enhancing the body's ability to heal. By relaxing the mind, hypnosis facilitates clarity of thoughts.

Hypnosis as a tool allows you to consciously access information at subconscious level. A voyage within is a fascinating experience and with proper guidance, the healing, the healing, the self understanding and the inner peace that follows is an homage to life itself, and for me as a hypnotherapist, a very humbling experience.

Hypnotherapy, using hypnosis to do therapy will be the subject of the next article.

Your Notes

Anny's Teaching

Hypnosis Vs. Hypnotherapy Part 2
What is the difference?

By Anny Slegten, Master Hypnotist, Clinical Hypnotherapist.

Consider a pencil. Depending what you want to use it for, you can choose a firm lead, a soft lead, or anything in between. You can write a report, fill out a form, write a poem or a love letter, doodle, make a schematic draw a portrait or a landscape.

The same goes for hypnosis. The way it is used depends on the training, the intentions and the ability of the person who uses it, and the need and level of cooperation of the person participating in the hypnotic experience. Therefore, I will only share my own views on the subject.

For me, hypnotherapy is usually regression therapy, going from effect back to cause, experiencing now the results of something that impressed our psyche before. How so? After all, are we not in the present, the now?

There is a part of us that remembers everything. As you are driving your car today, the way you are driving it now is the result of your interpretation of what you heard, observed and experienced as a passenger and a driver of a car from early childhood on. The same goes with our life.

We are the sum of our life experiences, and by regressing from effect back to cause, the fascinating voyages within our own consciousness usually bring a profound healing at a soul level, resulting in emotional order, clarity of thoughts, and inner peace.

Your Notes

Anny's Teaching

Hypnotherapy makes one also very much aware of how much thoughts can affect us physically. A common example is thinking of a lemon. Pretend you are holding it in your hand. Feel the texture, squeeze it, smell it, pretend you cut it in two crosswise, bring half a lemon to your mouth, and bite into it. Have you noticed how your body responded to this imaginary exercise?

The "Imaginary Lemon" experience partially explains why we all respond differently to situations experienced collectively: it is not what actually happened but what we perceive happened that makes an impact in our life. Emotionalized thoughts are like decisions frozen in time. Like ball-and-chain, these outdated decisions are mental blocks keeping attitudes to life at different stages of maturity.

Revisiting what happened allows us to have a new look at an old story, putting events in proper perspective, and making peace with ourselves. A most comforting, liberating experience.

Because of their inherent qualities, hypnosis and hypnotherapy can be used alone or in conjunction with other health care modalities. Enhancing other therapies, hypnosis and hypnotherapy can be powerful adjuncts to any therapy of your choice, restoring physical/emotional/mental balance. A great feeling.

Your Notes

Anny's Teaching

Outline For HYP #202 Practical Exam

PURPOSE:
Appropriately formulate and give a suggestion requested by client.

It is important to have the client's assistance at writing this script.

First ask the client if at the end of the recording they want to fall asleep or want to come back to 'now'.

1-TOGETHER WITH YOUR CLIENT, FORMULATE A SUGGESTION. Write it own.

2-LEAD THE CLIENT INTO A TRANCE. Remember the client will be alone when listening to this recording. Use an appropriated <u>spoken</u> induction.

3-SAY THE PRAYERS.

4-GIVE THE SUGGESTION <u>EXACTLY</u> AS FORMULATED.

5-DEEPEN THE TRANCE. Use an appropriated induction since the client will be alone.

6-GIVE THE SUGGESTION AGAIN, EXACTLY AS FORMULATED. By now, you may randomly choose and mix and match the written suggestion.

7-WRAP IT UP (CHOOSE FROM ANNY'S VERNACULAR).

STOP the recording if they want to fall asleep listening to the recording.

Your Notes

Anny's Teaching

8-BRING THE CLIENT BACK TO NOW (COMING OUT OF HYPNOSIS). And now, I am going to count from 1 to 5 etc.

9-POST-HYPNOTIC INTERVIEW:
What surprised you?
What did you learn?

www.success-and-more.com

Your Notes

Anny's Teaching

The Prayer

… and now, I am asking for our protection and wellbeing, and I say,

God, please allow only good things to come to (name) and me (name), the Hypnotherapist.

And for this blessing, we give thanks.

And now, you ask to be put into the protection of your Light, your very own Spark of Life. It is like a mini Sun in your chest. That light is the centre of your being. That light is you!

Concentrate on it, and let it shine, let it shine! Let is shine throughout every cell of your body, throughout your aura, cleansing your body, cleansing your aura, extending itself at one arm's length above you, beneath you, on each side of you, in front of you, and behind you, and mentally repeat with me:

"This is my body, this is my space,
only light can come to me,
only light can come from me,
only my light can be here."

Your Notes

Anny's Teaching

Coming Out Of Hypnosis

Now I'm going to count from one to five, and then I'll say:

"Your eyes are open and you are fully aware. You are rested, refreshed, relaxed, and feel wonderfully good."

- One, slowly, calmly, easily, and gently beginning to return to full awareness once again.

- Two, each muscle and nerve in your body is loose, limp and relaxed, and you feel wonderfully good.

- Three, from head to toe, you are feeling better in every way, physically better, mentally better, emotionally cool, calm, and serene.

- Four, your eyes begin to feel sparkling clean as if they were bathed in cool spring water.

- Five, eyelids open: you are fully aware. Take a good deep breath, fill up your lungs, open your eyes, and stretch.

Please note:

When working with a client that analyses everything, mix up the numbers to confuse the client. This will allow the work done to immediately go subconscious.

Your Notes

Anny's Teaching

Some Of Anny Slegten's Vernacular…

…inhale, exhale, sleep now.

When I say "sleep now", this is not the sleep you experience when you fall asleep: I am talking about the hypnotic sleep. This means, you relax completely your mind, and your body, so your subconscious mind, free of all restrain, is open and receptive to the suggestions you are receiving now...

…and **during this session** the sounds of my voice will make you go deeper and deeper into relaxation…

…and **during this session** each time the heating system is going on, and off, you will go twice as deep into relaxation…

…and we ask your subconscious mind, open and receptive to the suggestions you are receiving now, to sort all things out, and reveal to you whatever it feels you should know and understand about the issue that got you here today, and we ask your subconscious mind to reveal it to you in a gentle and most effective manner…

…and we ask your subconscious mind, open and receptive to the suggestions you are receiving now, to clear and resolve whatever should be cleared and resolved, and once it has been cleared and resolved, to let you know what has been cleared and resolved in a gentle and most effective manner and in a way that you understand, much to your surprise and delight.

www.success-and-more.com

Your Notes

Anny's Teaching

…and let an overwhelming feeling of tranquility flow all over you, and bless each member of your household, bless your family, bless your friends, bless your pets, if you have any – and that includes your house plants – bless your possession, bless your wishes, bless your light, the spark of life you have within you, and thank God, whoever you perceive God to be, for the good things of life…

…you are more relaxed than you have been for a while, and each time you enter this type of relaxation, you will enjoy a deeper and better state of relaxation, recharging your batteries, so to speak, physically, mentally, emotionally and spiritually, healing your life, healing your body, healing your soul …

…and we ask your subconscious mind, open and receptive to the suggestions you are receiving now, to make all the necessary improvements now, so that you this, or something better now manifests itself in your attitude, your behavior, your life, in a most successful, satisfying, diplomatic and joyful way, much to your surprise and delight…

…and for this blessing, we both give thanks …

Your Notes

Anny's Teaching

Additional New End Of Suggestions For End Of Sessions Or Recordings

Option 1: This Is Anny's Recent Mix And Match

Yes, (Name) _____, all is well.

That is right!

Only good things come to you.

From whatever happens always turns out in your favor.

That is right!

Love yourself into the future,

with pleasure, joy, comfort, ease, grace, and gratitude

and watch the magic fall out of the sky,

your heart (name) _____, full of love.

Your Notes

Anny's Teaching

Option 2: As Something Inside Of You Is About To Shift

I do not know what is about to shift.

You do not know what is about to shift.

All what I know is that something inside of you is about to shift.

As your subconscious mind, open and very receptive to the suggestions you are receiving now is sorting all things out.

And will reveal to you whatever it feels you should know and understand about the issue that got you here today.

And your subconscious mind will reveal it to you at most unexpected time, much to your surprise and delight.

Your Notes

Anny's Teaching

Option 3: The Following Is From Milton Erickson

At the end of the session to help your clients get out of their own way

I wonder how much you remember what I said seven minutes before (chose any length of time when applicable)

and your conscious mind can remember to forget or forget to remember whatever I said, the choice is yours.

And your subconscious mind will remember this and work in it, and it will be so.

I then add:

Much to your surprise and delight.

Your Notes

Anny's Teaching

Format For A Successful Practice

- **Interview** – approx. 15 minutes

  - To educate the therapist

- **Pre-Hypnotic Interview**

  - To educate the client

- **Lead The Person Into A Trance** (The Hypnotic process)

- **The Prayers**

- **The Hypnotic Process**

  - Access the feeling(s) attached to the issue
  - Review, update, transformation, and whatever is required
  - The resolution and healing process
  - Put the client back together so he/she feels solid inside
  - Conclusion and post-hypnotic suggestion
  - Bring the client back to now

- **Post-Hypnotic Interview**

  - What surprised you?
  - What have you learned?

Your Notes

Anny's Teaching

Wolberg's Arm Levitation

This context is done when the subject is already hypnotised

The subject is either stretched out on their back, on a couch or a bed or seated in a comfortable chair with their hands on their thighs, palms facing downward.

Muscle rehearsal

And you begin like this:
"I am going to count from one up to twenty.

As I do, a light, easy, pleasant feeling moves into your right hand and into your right arm.

As I continue counting, that feeling grows stronger and stronger.
Soon, you will feel the first slight movement, a slight movement of the fingers, a twitching of the muscles.

Then your hand begins to lift. It continues moving, lifting, and rising until it comes to rest up upon your body."

Now, at this point, take hold of the subject's wrist, and as you say,
"Your hand begins lift", *slowly begin to lift it.*
"Your hand begins lift", *continue lifting it,* "Until it comes to rest over on your body".
Move it over slowly and bring it down to rest upon their body.

That is called a muscle rehearsal.
It lets the subject know exactly what is expected.
Then place the hand down alongside their body again, with the palm facing downward and the fingers limply outstretched.
Then, take up from where you left off.

Your Notes

Anny's Teaching

You left off by saying, "Until it comes to rest over on your body".

"Now, when you feel the movement in your hand and in your arm, do not try to resist. You could resist if you chose to; That is not why you are here. Just let your subconscious mind do its perfect work.

Actual session

Alright now, we are ready to begin."

"Number one. The first light, easy sensation moves into the fingertips of your right hand."

"Number two. The feeling is spreading around beneath the fingernails."

"Number three. It is moving up to the first joint of the fingers."

"Number four. Spreading to the large knuckle across the back of the hand."

"Number five. The first slight movements begin to start taking place. Slight movements of the fingers and a twitching of the muscles."

"Number six. The light sensation spreads all across the back of your hand."

"Number seven. Spreading over and into your thumb."

"Number eight. Moving now all through the palm of your hand."

"Number nine. The light sensation spreads up and into your wrist."

"Think of your left hand now. You will see by comparison, your left hand is beginning to feel very, very heavy. While on number ten, your right hand grows lighter and lighter with each number I count; just a light as a feather floating in the breeze and even lighter. As light as a gas-filled balloon. Just as a gas-filled balloon will rise and float toward the ceiling,

Your Notes

Anny's Teaching

in the same way, by the time I reach the count of twenty, your right hand is moving, lifting, rising, and floating."

"Eleven. The light sensation has moved beyond your wrist now, spreading into your forearm."

"Number twelve and thirteen. Once again, think of your left hand. Your left hand has grown so heavy, it feels as though it were made of marble or stone."

"Fourteen. That light sensation is spreading up toward your elbow now."

"Fifteen. From the fingertips all the way up to the elbow, your hand has grown light, light and free, it's beginning to lift. It's moving, lifting, rising, and floating."

Now, at this point, you must gauge your suggestion to the kind of movement that you are getting. Sometimes you will begin to see the first twitching movements in the fingers and in the muscles on the third or fourth or fifth count. Sometimes you will have to go to ten or twelve or fifteen. If you see that you are not getting a response, stretch out the suggestions between your numbers and count more slowly. If, however, the yare responding rapidly, then speed up the tempo of your counting to keep pace with the speed their arm is lifting.

"Alright, sixteen. Now your arm is moving and lifting and rising. And as your arm is lifting, you're going deeper and deeper into hypnosis."

"Seventeen. Your hand continues moving, lifting, and rising until it comes to rest over on your body."

"Eighteen. Moving, lifting, rising, floating. Right on over now, and when your hand comes to rest upon your body, at that time your eyelids lock tightly closed. Your eyelids lock so tightly closed at that point, the more you try to open them, the tighter they're locking closed."

Your Notes

Anny's Teaching

"Nineteen. Your hand is getting ready to come down and rest upon your body."

"Number twenty. Now your hand has come to rest upon your body, and as it has, at the same time, your eyelids are locked so tightly closed, the more you try to open your eyelids, the tighter they're locking closed."

Now be sure to always use this phrasing. It is called the <u>Law of Reversed Mental Effect</u>. The suggestion is "try to open your eyelids." That is quite a different suggestion from "you cannot open your eyelids." Or, "It's impossible to open your eyelids." The word "try" implies failure. So, when you say, "Try to open your eyelids," that's suggestion number one. The second part of the suggestion is, "and find them locking tighter and tighter." So, it really means, "I want you to make an unsuccessful effort to open your eyelids. But I really want you to shut them more tightly closed when you make the effort." All right now, back to the suggestion to the subject.

"Alright now, try and satisfy yourself that your eyelids are indeed locked tightly closed. That's fine. Stop trying. Relax and go deeper in hypnosis."

Now again, at this point, it is very important that you do not try to satisfy yourself. Your purpose is to satisfy the subject. Do not say, "Try harder, harder than that. Oh, surely you are not trying hard enough." All they need to do is either make some kind of muscular effort to open the eyelids or allow about <u>three seconds</u> to go by without opening the eyelids. That is sufficient time for them to gain the realization that they did not open their eyelids. Now we will pyramid into and compound into the third suggestion.

"Alright now, stop trying. Just relax and go deeper into hypnosis. At the same time, your left arm has become so heavy, so heavy that it feels as though it were made of marble or stone or lead, and far too heavy to lift.

In fact, it seems as if your left arm were no longer under your control. In fact, your left arm feels so heavy that just the thought of it, the thought of

Your Notes

Anny's Teaching

lifting it, seems to be more than you want to deal with at this time. So, you may, if you wish, make an effort to lift your left arm. But, you find it just seems to weigh a ton.

All right, that is fine. Now just stop trying. Relax, and make no further effort. The feeling that you feel as your hand was lifting, that is the feeling of hypnosis. The feeling that you felt as your left arm seemed so heavy, that, too, is the feeling of hypnosis. The feeling that you felt as your eyelids seemed stuck or seemed not to want to open, that too is the feeling of hypnosis.

We call these responses the feeling of hypnosis because you realize, as well as I do, that there is no logical reason for your right arm to feel lighter than your left. There is no rational reason for your eyelids not to open when you wish to open them.

You see, the part of your mind that processes ideas, in terms of reason and rationality, is temporarily relaxed because you are now hypnotized. That means that you can accept ideas subconsciously, even ideas that are different from your previous experience, and that is what makes hypnosis valuable to you.

You might compare it to a stereo system. Usually, a stereo system has a balanced control. If you turn it to the right, you'll only hear the right speaker. Now, that does not mean the left speaker has been disconnected. It simply means, for the moment, it is inactive, and in the same way, when that critical factor of your conscious mind that processes the ideas according to their rationality and analyzes them and critically examines them, when that relaxes, you can accept and act upon ideas subconsciously. That is the nature of hypnosis.

So, in a moment, when I get you up, you are going to have a much clearer understanding of the dual nature of your conscious and subconscious mind. You will now know that you were not unconscious. You will know that you were not asleep. And yet, with the very nature of your experience, you will recognize what hypnosis truly is."

Your Notes

Anny's Teaching

"Alright now. I am going to count from one to five. At the count of five, I want you to let your eyelids open. You are then calm, rested, refreshed, relaxed, and you feel wonderfully good."

"One, slowly, calmly, easily and gently returning to your full awareness once again."

"Two, each muscle and nerve in your body is loose and limp and relaxed. You feel good."

"Three, from head to toe, you're feeling perfect in every way."

"On number four, your eyes begin to feel sparkling clear, just as though they were bathed in cold spring water. On the next number now, eyelids open, fully aware, feeling wonderfully good in every way."

"Number five, eyelids open now. You are fully aware once again. Take a good deep breath. Fill up your lungs and stretch."

Now wait, just for a moment, for the client to kind of orient himself to being up from hypnosis.

Then, say to him, "Well, you kind of surprised yourself, didn't you?"

Usually, they will answer "yes". *The moment they do, say,* "Tell me about it."

And let them begin to give you the feedback about how they feel about their experience.

If they say, "Well, what do you mean?" *or* "No, I was not surprised," *respond,* "Tell me how you felt when you felt your arm coming up. What kind of feeling was it when your eyelids did not seem to want to open? How did it feel to you when your left arm seemed so heavy?"

Now, through the use of these three tests, at this point you should have secured the conviction of the conscious mind for a recognition of the

Your Notes

Anny's Teaching

trance state, so that the client can leave your office from that first session, feeling either that they were indeed hypnotized, or at least confused. They are not sure whether or not they were hypnotized.

When they go home and they speak to someone else, when asked if they were hypnotized, the best that they can say is "Yes I was." "How do you know?" "Because of the way I behaved." The worst that they can say is, "Well, I'm not quite sure." And when they describe the behaviours of their arm lifting, or their eyelids sticking, or their left arm feeling heavy, that other person will assure them that they were indeed hypnotized.

This technique was named the Wolberg Arm Levitation in honour of Dr. Lewis Wolberg, medical psychiatrist.

Your Notes

Anny's Teaching

Direct Gaze Induction Technique

This is the most powerful technique of all, and also the most difficult to use because you have got to express perfect confidence. If you have any doubt, or hesitation, or fear, it will show in your eyes. The subject will read it and it will inhibit their response.

If the subject is standing,

you say to them, "Alright, I want you to fix your eyes right here."

Take your index finger out of your right hand and bring it under your right eye. If they are seated, say exactly the same thing, or if they are lying down on their back on a couch or on a bed, say exactly the same thing.

"Now I want you to look right here. Don not take your eyes from mine. Do not move or speak or nod your head or say "Uh huh" unless I ask you to. I know that you hear and understand me just as you know it. If you follow my simple instructions there is nothing in this world that can keep you from entering into a very deep and pleasant state of hypnosis and doing it in just a fraction of a second. Now, take a deep breath and fill up your lungs."

As you say this, take a deep breath yourself and take your right hand and move it in an upward motion in the air. Then say:

"Now exhale. That is fine, now a second and even deeper breath."

Now again bring up your hand. Exhale.

Let your hand come down. "Relax. Now a third deep breath."

Once again, hand up. "Exhale. Relax."

Your Notes

Anny's Teaching

Now raise your hand once again up over their head, about three feet in front of them, about two feet above their head with your index finger pointing out, just like you shake your finger at someone; hold it at an upraised position, at about a 45 degree angle, pointing it toward the ceiling.

Say to them: "And now, I am going to count from five down to one. As I do, your eyelids grow heavy, droopy, drowsy, and sleepy. By the time I reach the count of one, they close right down and you go deep in hypnotic slumber. Deeper than ever before."

"Alright, five, eyelids heavy, droopy, drowsy, and sleepy."

"Four, those heavy lids feel ready to close."

"Three, the next time you blink that's hypnosis coming on you then."

"Two, they begin closing, closing, closing, closing, closing, closing, closing, close them, close them, close them."

And at this point, as their eyelids begin to flutter and close, you stand with <u>your hand on their shoulder</u>, move it around behind their head with a gentle pressure,

say: "They're closing, closing, closing, closing. One, <u>sleep now</u>."

Pull their head forward. Say,

"Now, just relax and go deeply into hypnosis, deeper than you've ever been before."

Now when you are looking the subject in the eye, it's important for you not to blink. You can learn the direct gaze by practising in the mirror. Learn to narrow your eyes slightly, not enough to look ludicrous or funny, but enough to keep your eyeball from drying out, because that is really what causes blinking. You blink to moisten that eyeball because the fluid keeps evaporating from it. Now, also, just as in the arm

Your Notes

Anny's Teaching

levitation, time your numbers in response to what you see happening in the subject's eyes.

When you say, Five, eyelids heavy, droopy, drowsy, and sleepy,"

you may see that you just don not feel any quality or response. Then stretch out your suggestion a little bit.

You say, "Five, eyelids heavy, droopy, drowsy, and sleepy, your eyelids feel so heavy; four, your heavy lids begin to feel as though they are getting ready to close; three, the very next time they blink, that's a hypnosis coming on you then."

Now, suddenly, you see them beginning to blink. And then you say,

"And now they begin closing, closing,"

and you pick up the tempo. Follow your pattern, your tempo, with what you see happening with the subject.

Now the direct gaze technique is the most effective because all of the imagery associated with hypnosis, all of the ideas that the person has learned from the movies, novels, cartoons, and comic strips, all show that the hypnotist's eyes have power.

It is also in mythology. On the back of your dollar bill, right above the pyramid on the left side, you will see the image of the all powerful eye of God.

Your Notes

Anny's Teaching

Hands Closing Together

From: Gil Boyne

This is an extraordinarily effective technique and it has been used by a great many of my graduates as their favourite induction. Although you can do this with the client lying on their back and their arms extending upward toward the ceiling or standing in front of them and having them extend their arms toward you, the best position is to have your client seated in a chair. Stand in front of them, about six feet distant, extend both of your arms out towards them, with the palms of your hands facing each other, your fingers held together, your thumbs pointing upward and speak to them in this manner:

"Extend both of your arms out in front of you like this … stiffen your arms; lock your elbows; palms of your hands facing each other; your thumbs up; your fingers together. Now in a moment I am going to bring my finger in between your hands. Until I do, I want you to look right here into my eyes; keep looking at me. Just as soon as I bring my index finger in between your two hands, take your eyes from mine and fix them on my fingertips; then I will move my finger. When I do, do not move your eyes, keep looking straight ahead between your hands."

"Alright, now bring your eyes down here to my fingertips. Now I am going to move my finger, and when I do, do not move your eyes. Keep looking straight ahead between your hands. Then, as I count from three down to one, close your eyelids down. Now, the very moment that your eyelids close down, your two hands begin drawing together. Just imagine there is a magnet on the palm of each hand which is drawing them in closer, closer, closing and moving in until your two hands touch."

Your Notes

Anny's Teaching

Now, as you say this to the client, when you reach that point where you say, "The very moment your eyelids close down, your two hands begin closing," you must grasp their hands *and slowly as you say "closing, closing, closing," you will slowly push them together. That again is the* muscle rehearsal *so that they know what they are expected to do, and how they are expected to behave.*

Then, separate their hands again and say, "Alright, when I count from three down to one, close your *eyelids* down." *And at this point, position your hands; each of your hands under each of their hands with your index finger pointed outward. And, as you begin to count from three down to one for them to close their eyelids down, you begin* sweeping your fingers *in toward the center, so that the last thing they see visually are your hands moving toward each other. So, you say:*

"Alright, three, two, one, close your eyelids down." *And as you say* "Close your eyelids down"; *you are sweeping your two hands toward each other.*

"Alright, now they are closing, closing, closing, closing, closing, closing, closing, closing and almost touching, closing and almost touching."

"Picture the magnet in the palm of your hand. They are closing and moving in, closing and moving in. They are closing, closing, closing, closing, closing, closing and moving in, moving in and closing, closing and moving in, moving in and closing, closing, closing and moving in, moving in and closing, until your two hands touch. They are closing and almost touching. Picture the magnets in the palm of each hand as they are closing, closing and moving in."

Now watch for the movement. You see their hands coming in closer and closer. Wait until they have covered at least half the distance. Then say this:

Your Notes

Anny's Teaching

"The moment your two hands touch, a wave of relaxation will move all across your body. The moment you feel your two hands touch, every muscle and every nerve in your body will completely relax. All right now, they are closing, closing, almost touching, closing, closing, closing, closing and almost touching, closing and almost touching, closing and almost touching, closing and almost touching. Now they are touching. Let your head come forward on your chest; let your arms drop limply into your lap; let every muscle and every nerve now grow loose and limp and relaxed and feel good all over now."

Now, you might add one other thing. As you are giving the suggestion, "You hands are closing, closing, closing, closing and almost touching," *and as you see they are about to touch, just as they are touching, take your hands, put them on the back of their hands and press them together and say*, "Now sleep." *And with a steady pull, kind of pull their hands down into their lap and say,* "Let your head come forward on your chest and continue going easily, pleasantly, fully into a wonderfully pleasant state of hypnotic relaxation." *Then, just continue with your suggestion.*

Now you may use this as a suggestibility test so that when their hands come together, you simply say, "Open your eyes; well you kind of surprised yourself, did you not? Were you surprised to feel your hands closing together?"

Then, be quiet and listen to their feedback. If, however, you are going to bypass the suggestibility test and use it as an induction, just the very instant that their hands close, that is when you say, "Now sleep." Pull their hands in a slow, steady pull or push them down into their lap, if you wish, you might want to just put your hand behind their neck and gently pull their head forward. Immediately check for the limpness in the arms and continue with your deepening procedures.

Your Notes

Anny's Teaching

From Janice Letourneau, January 28, 1995

Phantom Limbs

1. Create a visual identification of the phantom limb and the phantom pain. Be sure that you allow the client to choose his/her own picture.

2. Ensure the client has an intellectual understanding of the phenomenon along with the suggestion that pain will be gone as soon as the nerves understand that the limb is gone.

3. Give the client control over the phantom limb by the use of exercise and make it fun.

4. Once the client fully accepts that he/she has full control of both the phantom limb and the phantom pain the client will dispose of it when the client is ready.

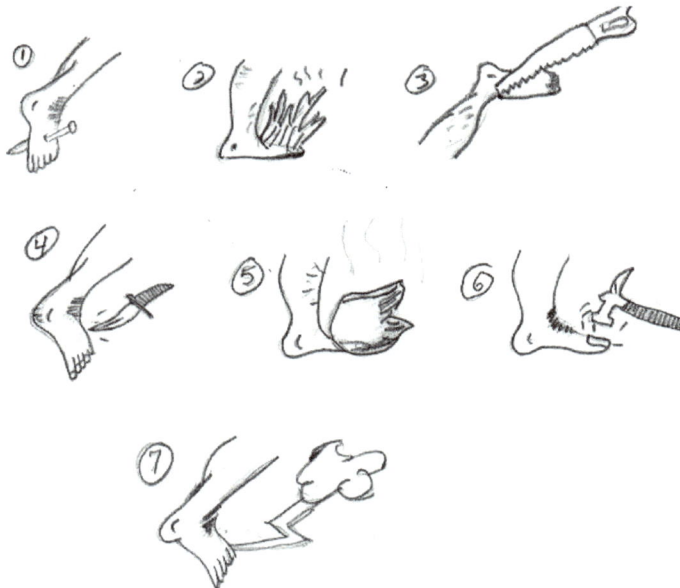

5.

Artwork k courtesy of Brad Letourneau

Your Notes

Anny's Teaching

Sticky Fingers Induction

Please make yourself as comfortable as possible. Remove your eyeglasses, loosen clothing that binds you in any way, and remove your shoes if they are tight.

Play Music

And now, stare at the thumb and middle finger of your writing hand.

Put them together and imagine they are glued tightly.

Push them together and imagine they are also bound with strong adhesive tape.

The glue is drying, and the finger and thumb are stuck tightly together.

Stare at them and imagine they are becoming stuck tighter and tighter.

And now, count from <u>five</u> down to <u>one</u>, and after each count, say "Stuck tighter".

When you get down to <u>one</u>, they will be stuck so tightly you will feel they are stuck, no matter how hard you try to pull them apart.

All right.

Keep staring at your thumb and middle finger of your writing hand and start counting from five down to one, and after each count, say "<u>Stuck tighter</u>"

Five, stuck tighter …

Four, stuck tighter …

Your Notes

Anny's Teaching

Three, stuck tighter …

Two, stuck tighter …

One, stuck tighter …

It feels that the harder you try to pull them apart, the more tightly they will stick together.

Keep staring at the thumb and the middle finger of your writing hand.

If you keep thinking this one thought to the exclusion of all others, you will be unable to pull your thumb and middle finger apart.

If you deviate and think "I'll bet I could pull them apart if I wanted to", your mind has wandered from the original thought and you are not following instructions.

Think they are stuck, and they will remain stuck.

Close your eyes.

You will keep your eyes closed until I ask you to open them.

And as I say this, you can easily separate your fingers.

Take a deep breath.

As you exhale, imagine all tension leaving your body.

Take a deep breath.

And as you exhale, all tension is leaving your body.

And as you take another deep breath, and exhale, you feel more and more relaxed … … …

Your Notes

Anny's Teaching

Dave Elman Technique Of Induction

Hand Closing

Explaining what will be done:

For the moment, rest your arms limply on your thighs, just like this. Now, I want you to out here at my hand. In a moment I am going to bring my hand up in front of your eyes like this. When I do, I will pass my hand down in front of your eyes.

Keep your eyes fixed on my little finger.

As I pass my hand down, that will cause your eyelids to close down.

The process:

"All right, now fix your eyes on my little finger."

"Now, I am passing my hand down in front of your eyes, and as I do, let your eyelids close down."

"Now your eyelids are close down."

"I want you to relax every tiny muscle and nerve in and around your eyelids."

"I want you to relax them so much that they would not work even if wanted them to do so."

"Now, when you know that you have relaxed them that much, they would not work if you wanted them to. Test them, you will see you have been completely successful. You relaxed them that much that would not work if you wanted them to."

Your Notes

Anny's Teaching

Now, test them. You will see you have been completely successful.

(Pause three seconds)

"All right. That is fine. Now, stop trying and just relax and go deeper now."

Your Notes

Anny's Teaching

Hand Dropping

"Now, I am going to raise your hand. I will do it by grasping your right thumb in my fingers like this."

As I lift your hand, just let it hang, kind of limply in my hand then, when I drop it, let it drop like a wet limp dish rag.

"When your hand touches your body, as it drops, I want you to send a wave of relaxation from the top of your head all the way down to the tips of your toes. That will double your present level of relaxation."

"Now, I am raising your hand. Just let it hang into mine. That is it. Let it hang limply. I have got it now. Just turn it loose there."

"That is good. Now, when I drop it, let it drop like a wet dish rag, and as it touches your body, send a wave of relaxation from the top of your head down to the tip of your toes."

That is fine!

"Now, we will do that again with the left hand. I am going to pick up your left hand, and as I take your thumb, let it hang limply in my hand."

"That is good. Now you are getting the idea."

"When I drop it, let it drop like a limp wet dish rag. When it touches your body, send a wave of relaxation from the top of your head to the tip of your toes and double the present level of relaxation."

"That is fine!"

Your Notes

Anny's Teaching

100 – Deeper Asleep

"Now, your body is relaxed, and I am going to show you how to relax your mind."

"Listen carefully."

"The next time I touch your forehead, I want you to begin counting from one hundred backward in this way:"

"One hundred, deeper asleep,
Ninety-nine deeper asleep.
Ninety-eight, deeper asleep.
And so on."

"After counting just a few numbers, by the time you reach ninety-seven, or ninety-six. At the most ninety-five, you will find the numbers disappearing."

"You will find your mind has become so relaxed that you will just relax them out of your mind."

"All right. Get ready now."

Your Notes

Anny's Teaching

Three, two, one (Tap the forehead), ***begin counting.***

"One hundred, deeper asleep. Good, slow them down now.
Ninety-nine, deeper asleep. Good.
Ninety-eight, deeper asleep. Fine.
Ninety-seven," start relaxing them out of your mind, deeper asleep.
Ninety-six," let them start disappearing and fading, deeper asleep.
Ninety-five, deeper asleep," let them relax out of your mind now.
Ninety-four, deeper asleep". Now let them fade away completely."

"That is fine.
You have relaxed your body.
You have relaxed your mind.
You have gone into a much deeper state of hypnosis."

Your Notes

Anny's Teaching

Hand Drop Instant Induction

Explain to the person standing or sitting in front of you

Put your hand on mine.

When I count to four, press down as hard as you can.

One, stare at my fingers *(Holding your fingers of your other hand in front of the person to create eye fatigue).*

Two, pressing down harder. Press it down harder.

Three, eyelids heavy, droopy, feeling drowsy and sleepy.

Four, *(In a <u>rapid and unexpected</u> movement, bring your fingers down and pull your hand away from under the person's and command)* "SLEEP"

Your Notes

Anny's Teaching

Instant Rapid Induction

Remember: Hypnosis is simply the bypass of the critical factor of the conscious mind and the establishment of acceptable selective thinking.

1.   Create a rapid unexpected movement of some part or all of the client's body. This creates the bypass of the critical Factor by overloading the nervous system.

To the subject, standing in front of you:
Stand facing me. That is right. Now step forward.
(Place your right hand on the person's head, supporting the base of the skull grasp the person's right arm at elbow with your left hand).

Bring your feet closer together. Closer. That is right. Breathe in deeply.

2. *Fire in the suggestion* "SLEEP" *as the persons breathes out,* ***(with a sudden forward pulling movement of the hands, lightly jerk the subject towards you).***

3. ***(If the person's legs begin to buckle say)*** Your legs are strong beneath you, and you can stand and sleep!

Your Notes

Anny's Teaching

Escalator Induction

By Janice Letourneau

Imagine yourself standing at the top of an escalator. At the bottom is a place where you **feel** safe, warm and comfortable, totally at peace with yourself and your surroundings. As I count you will go down the escalator and deeper into relaxation.

20 - Step on the escalator. You are able to **listen** to and concentrate on my voice easily and totally. Easily and gently go deeply relaxed.

19 – As you go down, look at the beauty around you. Notice how the **sights** make you relax twice as much.

18, 17 – As you go down, hear the **sounds** around you. Notice how the sounds make you relax.

16, 15, 14 – As you go down, **smell** the fresh air. Notice how the smell makes you relax.

13, 12, 11 – As you go down, **feel** the tension leave your mind and your body.

10, 9, 8 – You are experiencing a very pleasant feeling of increased awareness and sensitivity throughout your consciousness.

7, 6, 5 – As your mind and body are relaxed, a magnificent feeling of peace, relaxation and joy flows throughout your body, relaxing your muscles, relaxing your emotions, relaxing your nerves and relaxing your mind.

Your Notes

Anny's Teaching

4, 3, 2 – The air is comfortable to breathe. So, you breathe deeply, and every breath carries you deeper and deeper into relaxation.

1 – Step off the escalator and into your safe place. Find a comfortable place to sit and relax. Notice how warm and how comfortable and how safe you are.

Your Notes

Anny's Teaching

Waterfall Induction

By Rachel Hall

Together, with your co-operation, we are going to create your very own space. A place where every **sound, sight, taste, smell,** and **touch** manifests itself into incredible happiness and peaceful relaxation. A place where you pamper yourself, a place just for you and only you.

Now, imagine your place. Concentrate on the size, it can be as big or as small as you like. This is your place, make it fit you.

Notice how your place looks, how it reflects yourself. Become aware of how it makes you feel knowing that very soon everything is going to fall perfectly into place. Notice how you are already becoming more deeply relaxed and falling deeper into that lovely state of altered awareness which is hypnosis.

And now, find a place for a beautiful set of curtains and put them there. These curtains are long, so long they touch the floor or the ground, whichever the case may be.

Now these curtains are about to reveal to you what exactly makes this place of yours so special.

As you stare at the top of the curtains, **watch** as the pleats begin to look like they are falling out. They resemble water, and by the time you move your eyes slowly from the top of the curtain down, it has changed into a wonderful waterfall.

Feel a spray as the water crashes at the bottom. As you notice how cool it is on your skin, you go deeper into relaxation.

Your Notes

Anny's Teaching

Listen to the **sound** the water makes, notice how this sound carries you deeper into your trance.

Go to your waterfall, cup your hands and take a sip of the water. **Taste** how fresh, clean, and cool it is and go deeply relaxed.

Now, take a deep breath and **smell** the humidity in the air, and this doubles your present level of relaxation.

This is your place to come back to whenever you feel the want. This is your place to imagine anything you wish. And this place is very special because imagination is the only thing that can change a curtain into a waterfall. You are a very powerful person, and you can make anything you wish come true.

Your Notes

Anny's Teaching

Script For A Good Night Sleep

Suggestion for a good night sleep usually given at the end of a session:

…as you are going deeper and deeper into relaxation, enjoy the feeling that is becoming so familiar to you,

And tonight, and every night, when you are ready to fall asleep with your head on your pillow, remember how relaxed you felt, remember being in this (my) chair, remember the sound of my voice, and then, take a deep breath, and as you exhale you will close your eyes and go into a wonderful slumber, to wake up a minute or two before waking up time, getting up, feeling refreshed, relaxed, renewed, rejuvenated, at peace with yourself and with the world around you, ready for good day.

Your Notes

Anny's Teaching

A Post-Hypnotic "Self" Re-Induction Technique

This is a very good technique to have a new client conditioned at going into a trance.

When a client has been hypnotized before, ask the client to describe how the "other" person/hypnotist induced the trance.

As your client describes it, notice how they are "talking themselves" into a trance.

Then, go through your own hypnotic induction technique whatever method you choose (since the client does not know they put themselves into a trance and expect you to do it….)

NOW YOUR CLIENT IS IN A TRANCE AND READY FOR THE WORK THEY CAME FOR.

www.success-and-more.com

Your Notes

Anny's Teaching

Practice

A Post-Hypnotic "Self" Re- Induction Technique And Suggestion for A Good Night Sleep

This is a very good technique to have a new client conditioned at going into a trance. When a client has been hypnotized before, ask the client to describe how the "other person/hypnotist induced the trance.

Trance Induction

As your client describes it, notice how your client is "talking themselves" into a trance. Then, go through your own hypnotic induction technique (since the clients do not know they put themselves into a trance and expect you to do it….)

Prayer

Deepen the trance – choosing your own method.

Give the following sleep suggestion:

…as you are going deeper and deeper into relaxation, enjoy the feeling that is becoming so familiar to you…

And tonight, and every night, when you are ready to fall asleep with your head on your pillow, remember how relaxed you felt, remember being this (my) chair, remember the sound of my voice, and then, take a deep breath, and as you exhale you will close your eyes and go into a wonderful slumber, to wake up a minute or two before waking up time, feeling refreshed, relaxed, renewed, rejuvenated, at peace with yourself and with

Your Notes

Anny's Teaching

the world around you, and with the world around you, getting up and ready for a very good day.

Deepen the trance again – choosing your own method.

Bring the client back to now (coming out of hypnosis).

Post hypnotic interview:

What surprised you?
What have you learned?

Your Notes

Anny's Teaching

The Suggestion Loop

The idea is to create a gear with each tooth of the gear bearing a suggestion.

When one of the suggestions is accepted at subconscious level, the complete gear is caught in the system and all the suggestions are accepted.

Example:

From this point on:

The more you have the pleasure of having physical, mental, emotional, spiritual & financial focus and clarity, **the more** you enjoy completing your hypnosis and hypnotherapy certificate.

The more you enjoy completing your hypnosis and hypnotherapy certificate, **the more** you have the pleasure of writing, reviewing, editing, & publishing your book.

The more you have the pleasure of writing, reviewing, editing, & publishing your book, **the better** your focus to carry on your life purpose.

The better your focus to carry on your life purpose, **the better** you follow your path to true happiness to fulfillment.

The better you follow your path to true happiness to fulfillment, **the more** you have the pleasure of having physical, mental, emotional, spiritual & financial focus and clarity.

The more you have the pleasure of having physical, mental, emotional, spiritual & financial focus and clarity, **the more** you enjoy completing your hypnosis and hypnotherapy certificate.

Your Notes

Anny's Teaching

Hypnosis Before Surgery

Example of the use of a recording for the benefit of the client.

Anny:

Okay, please make yourself as comfortable as possible. Loosening clothing that binds you in any way and remove your shoes if they are tight.

Now that you are comfortable, listen very closely to my voice and follow suggestions. With your cooperation, you will have the most pleasant experience. Feeling refreshed, relaxed, renewed, rejuvenated. At peace with yourself and with the world around you.

And as you take a slow deep breath and exhale, become aware of your lungs. Your lungs. They are expanding and contracting, expanding and contracting in a beautiful rhythmic manner. And every breath that you take makes you go deeper and deeper into relaxation. And as your breath flows, as it comes, as it goes, notice that the sensation is a little cooler when you breath in than when you breath out. Just a little cooler. Just a little cooler. That breath of your's. In your mind, follow it, as it goes within you, bringing you life and good health. Follow it, as you take a slow deep breath. As you exhale, notice how it exchanged good health and exhale whatever has to be cleared.

And as you follow your breath, thank it. Thank your breath and feel the flow of life as you breath in and as you breath out. And let all your cares fade away, fade away, fade away. And as you are relaxing more and more, welcome that feeling of relaxation that becomes so familiar to you. Such a familiar feeling. So just relax. Trust the flow of life.

As I am asking for your protection and your well-being and I say God, please allow only good things to come to us, and for this blessing, we give thanks.

Your Notes

Anny's Teaching

And now, you ask to be placed into the protection of your very own light. Your very own light, your spark of life. It is like a mini sun inside your chest. Some people can see it. Some people can feel it. Some people simply know it is there. That light of yours.

That very beautiful light of yours. Let it shine, let it shine. Let it shine throughout every cell of your body. Throughout your aura. Cleansing your body. Cleansing your aura. Strengthening your body. Strengthening your aura. Expanding itself at one arm's length above you, beneath you, at each side of you, in front of you and behind you.

And mentally repeat with me, this is my body, and this is my space. Only light can come to me. Only light can come from me. Only my light can be here.

Contemplate that light of yours. That light. Spark of light. That light of yours. That is part of the universe. That light of yours, makes you part of the Universe. Contemplate it. And as you contemplate it, you feel more and more relaxed.

You know how you want to be. You want to be comfortable in your body from the top of your head to the tip of your toes. That is right and you know the decision you made, so it is so.

You want to be at all times comfortable in your body from the top of your head to the tip of your toes. Contemplate what you want. Contemplate how you want to be, which is the reason for your decision and trust your decision. Trust also the system that will help you get there.

So keep in mind the results and the more you keep in mind the results, the more and more you feel comfortable with yourself and with the world around you. The more you feel comfortable, feeling really at peace with yourself and with the world around you. That is right. As you go deeper and deeper and deeper into relaxation.

Your Notes

Anny's Teaching

So as you take a slow deep breath and exhale, find yourself at a place that suggests relaxation to you. Find yourself there. And as you are at that place that suggests relaxation to you, relax, relax, relax, and trust your decisions. Trust the people who will help you obtain what you want and most of all trust also that light of yours. That light of yours.

So relax, relax and that light of yours, become very much aware of it and notice that the part of you, that light is connected to the Universe, and as you follow the stream of light, you will connect with a Being in the light that is very important to you.

Connect with that Being that is in the light. That is right. And as you take a slow deep breath and exhale, explain to that Being of light how you want to be. How you want to feel about your decision, the decision that you made so that you feel comfortable in your body from the top of your head to the tip of your toes.

And as you are connecting with that Being that is into the light, pay attention to the music being played at the moment and tell yourself that each crystal sound is from a star and that the crystal sounds are reassuring you, reminding you that you are part of that Universe and to relax. And as you are listening to the sounds coming from the stars, the crystal sounds are suggestions to you to relax, be cool, calm and collected.

Trust your decision. Trust the people who are helping you at obtaining what you want to be. At obtaining how you want to feel in your body. How you want life to be for you. Comfortable, pleasant, enjoyable at all times and you want to experience that pleasantness from the top of your head to the tip of your toes.

So just relax, relax, relax, and let all your cares fade away, fade away, fade away, fade away. As you go deeper and deeper and deeper into relaxation. Deeper and deeper. Deeper and deeper and deeper into relaxation. Letting all your cares fade away, fade away, fade away. Trusting your decision. Trusting the people that will help you at feeling in your body the way you want to feel. Trusting the Universe also. So just relax.

Your Notes

Anny's Teaching

Listen to the crystal sounds. The sounds coming from the stars. Singing for you. Reminding you that you are part of the Universe and feeling great about it. So just relax, relax, relax, and let all your cares fade away, fade away, fade away, fade away.

You know that some experiences are not very pleasant, and you know also as you are reviewing all your experiences that were not that pleasant, it always ended in a very pleasant way. All of it. So, trust your decision. Now, everything will turn out the way you like it to be. It happened before and it will happen this time again.

So, trust life, trust life. As you go deeper and deeper and deeper into relaxation, and during this experience, every familiar sound that you hear makes you go deeper and deeper into a wonderful state of relaxation and when you are relaxed like that, you are allowing your body to regulate itself to good health, enjoying a sharp mind, a clear head, and a tranquil heart. That is right. Enjoying a sharp mind, a clear head, and a tranquil heart.

So listen to the stars. They are singing for you and with each crystal sound you are going deeper and deeper and deeper into relaxation. That's right and project yourself a few weeks from now and in your mind's eye see yourself smiling, feeling so great. That is right.

See yourself in a few weeks from now happy, relaxed, very happy and relaxed. Feeling great from the top of your head to the tip of your toes, feeling totally at peace with yourself. Totally, totally at peace with yourself.

So, relax, relax, relax. That is right, Relax and each time you want to relax and feel at peace with yourself, in your mind you will hear the stars singing. You are part of the Universe. And as you are becoming aware of your light, just smile at the thought that you are a star too. You are a star among the stars.

Your Notes

Anny's Teaching

So just relax and at the end of this recording all what you have to do is take a slow deep breath and as you exhale, you will go into a wonderful slumber. To come back to full awareness a minute or two before waking up time, feeling refreshed, relaxed, renewed rejuvenated. Totally, totally at peace with yourself and with the world around you.

So just relax and as you take a slow deep breath again, and exhale, see yourself a few weeks from now, smiling. Feeling great, feeling so happy, so happy. Happy with your decisions. That is right. Happy, very, very happy of your decisions. So relax, trust that light of yours. Listen to the stars sing for you. You are part of them, and they are part of you.

And into that light, there is someone that you trust that is there also, looking after you, making sure that the result of your decision is exactly what you want. So listen to the stars. Listen to the stars. Listen as you go deeper and deeper and deeper into relaxation. Deeper and deeper into relaxation. Trusting your judgment, trusting your decision, trusting the people that are helping you in that decision. You know you are in good hands. You know you are in very, very good hands. Connect with that Being that is in the light and realize that you are in very good hands.

So relax and project yourself a few weeks from now and notice how good you feel. Notice how happy you feel and notice also how comfortable you feel from the top of your head to the tip of your toes. That is right. So relax, relax, relax, relax. That is right, just relax and trust your light. Trust it.

As you go deeper and deeper and deeper into relaxation, trust that light of yours. Trust your decisions and trust life. That is right and at the end of this recording, you will take a slow deep breath and as you exhale, you will go in a much, much deeper state of relaxation.

Your Notes

Anny's Teaching

Going into a wonderful slumber. To wake up a minute or two before wake up time, feeling refreshed, relaxed, renewed, rejuvenated, totally, totally at peace with yourself and with the world around you. That is right. Totally, totally at peace with yourself and with the world around you.

So relax, relax, relax.

(deep breath).

The stars are singing for you. The stars are singing for you. You are part of them, and they are part of you.

Your Notes

Anny's Teaching

Consciousness

The subconscious mind is highly suggestible as long as the suggestion is presented in such a way that it makes sense to the conscious mind **or** matches the desire at subconscious level ((usually a belief) That is the reason that sometimes it works right away, sometimes it takes some work to get there.

Therefore:

*Hypnosis as "an altered state of consciousness in which the subconscious mind **can be** highly suggestible".*

When in a state of shock, in a coma or anaesthetized , a person <u>loses consciousness</u> everything said or perceived lodges at subconscious level.

Hypnosis is a manipulation of the mind who then goes into a   trance and <u>is still conscious</u>.

Your Notes

Anny's Teaching

Brain Waves – Information

DELTA   Deep Sleep
0.5 to 3 cycles/seconds

THETA   Trance, drowsiness, or light sleep
4 to 8 cycles per second

ALPHA   Relaxed wakefulness or light sleep
8 to 14 cycles per second

BETA   Active everyday consciousness
14 to 35 cycles per second

Voltage between head and other parts of the body become more negative during physical activity, decline in sleep and reverse to positive under general anaesthesia.

It is a change in voltage.

Information from:
The Body Electric
By Roberts O. Becker, MD and Gary Selden

Your Notes

Anny's Teaching

www.success-and-more.com

www.success-and-more.com

www.success-and-more.com

www.success-and-more.com

www.success-and-more.com

www.success-and-more.com

www.success-and-more.com

www.success-and-more.com

www.success-and-more.com

www.success-and-more.com

www.success-and-more.com

www.success-and-more.com

www.success-and-more.com

www.success-and-more.com

www.success-and-more.com

www.success-and-more.com

www.success-and-more.com

www.success-and-more.com

www.success-and-more.com

www.success-and-more.com

www.success-and-more.com

www.success-and-more.com

www.success-and-more.com

www.success-and-more.com

www.success-and-more.com

www.success-and-more.com

www.success-and-more.com

www.success-and-more.com

www.success-and-more.com

www.success-and-more.com

www.success-and-more.com

www.success-and-more.com

www.success-and-more.com

www.success-and-more.com

www.success-and-more.com

www.success-and-more.com

www.success-and-more.com

www.success-and-more.com

www.success-and-more.com

www.success-and-more.com

www.success-and-more.com

www.success-and-more.com

www.success-and-more.com

www.success-and-more.com

www.success-and-more.com

www.success-and-more.com

www.success-and-more.com

www.success-and-more.com

www.success-and-more.com

Online Store, Contact, and More…

You may contact Anny by visiting any of her websites and scroll down the home page to the contact information.

http://www.annyslegten.com
Anny's private website and online store.

http://www.success-and-more.com
To find the description of the many services offered, and more.

http://www.htialberta.com
The Hypnotism Training Institute of Alberta including descriptions of hypnosis and hypnotherapy courses given.

http://www.reiki-canada.com
About the Reiki Training Centre of Canada.

http://www.slegtenianhypnosis.com
Although open to anyone interested in this fascinating hypnosis modality, this website information is for graduates of the Hypnotism Training Institute of Alberta.

http://www.connectwithanny.com
This is the best place to keep up to date with Anny – including seeing all her latest books and how to order them on Amazon.

Other books by Anny Slegten…

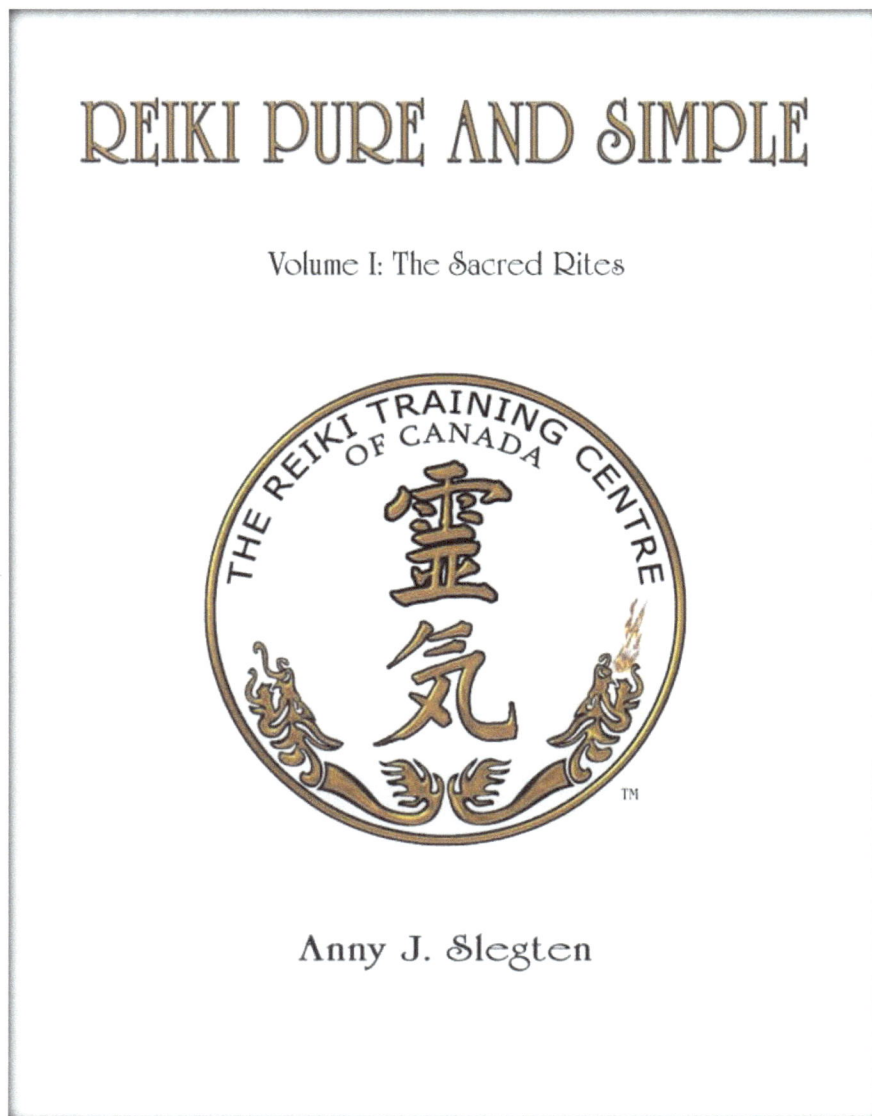

REIKI PURE AND SIMPLE

Volume I: The Sacred Rites

THE REIKI TRAINING CENTRE
OF CANADA

霊
気

Anny J. Slegten

Reiki Training Centre of Canada
Class Material
http://www.reiki-canada.com

REIKI PURE AND SIMPLE

Volume II: Reiki Ryoho Hikkei
(The Most Important Methods for Reiki)

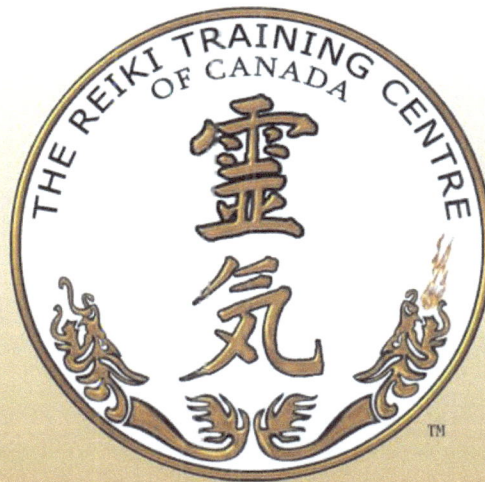

THE REIKI TRAINING CENTRE
OF CANADA

霊気療法必携

Anny J. Slegten

This book is a must read for Reiki Practitioners
regardless of their spiritual lineage
and could be of great benefit to Energy Healers
http://www.reiki-canada.com

REIKI PURE AND SIMPLE

Volume III: The Many Ways of Reiki

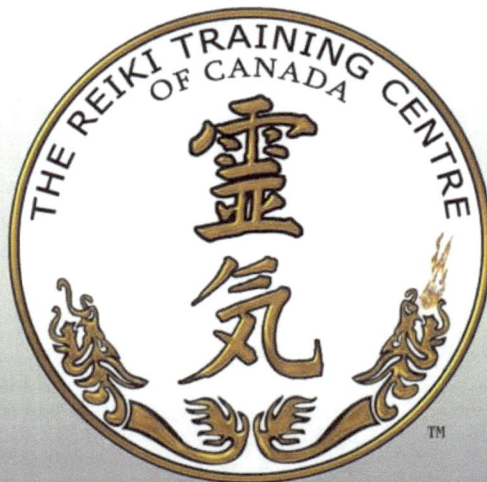

Anny J. Slegten

The Many Ways of Reiki
http://www.reiki-canada.com

www.success-and-more.com

REIKI PURE AND SIMPLE

TRADITIONAL JAPANESE REIKI

Volume IV: The Teacher Manual

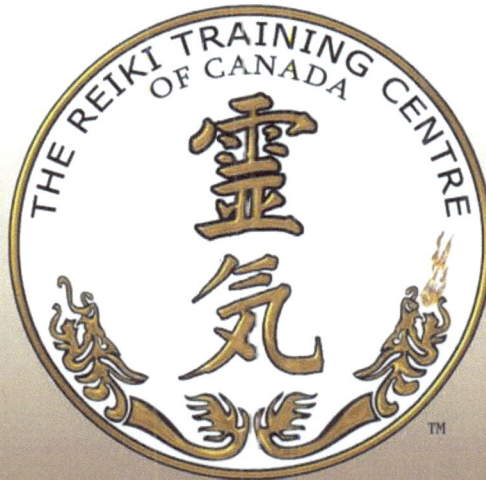

THE REIKI TRAINING CENTRE OF CANADA

靈氣

Anny J. Slegten

The Reiki Training Centre of Canada
Teacher's Manual
http://www.reiki-canada.com

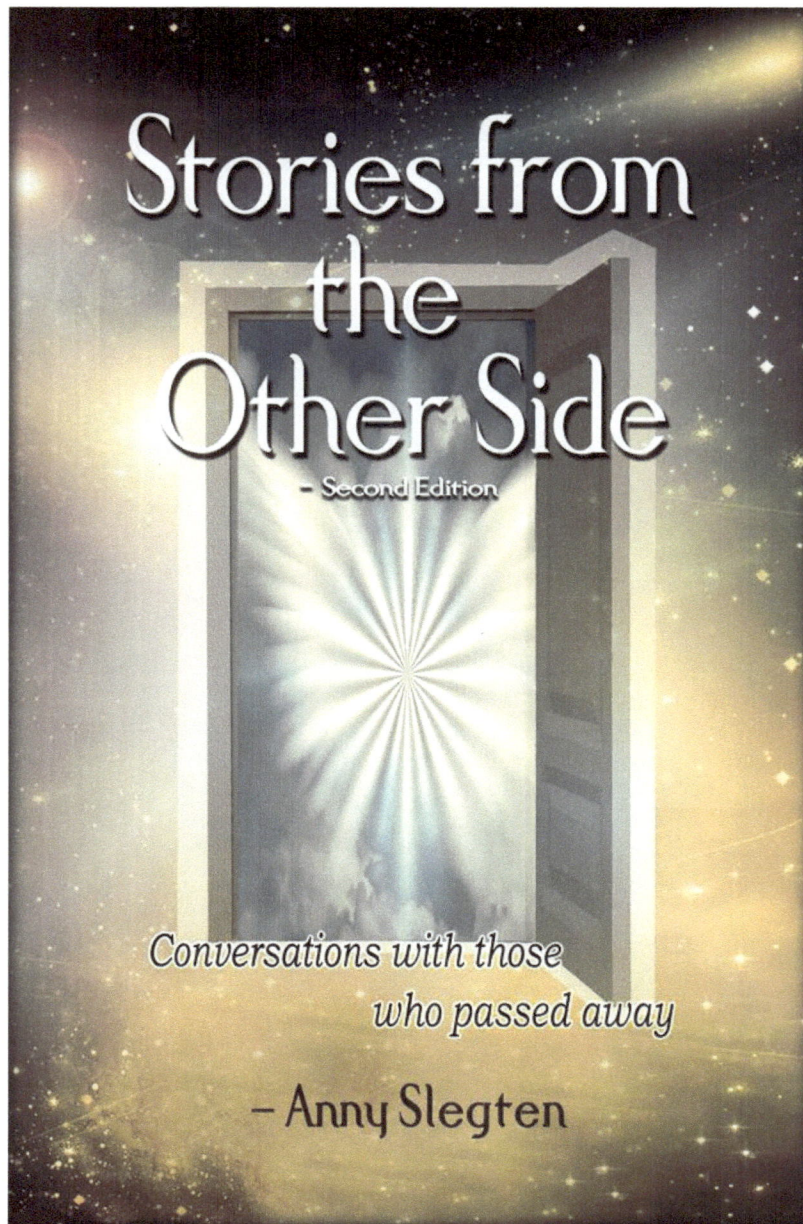

Stories from The Other Side – Second Edition
http://www.connectwithanny.com

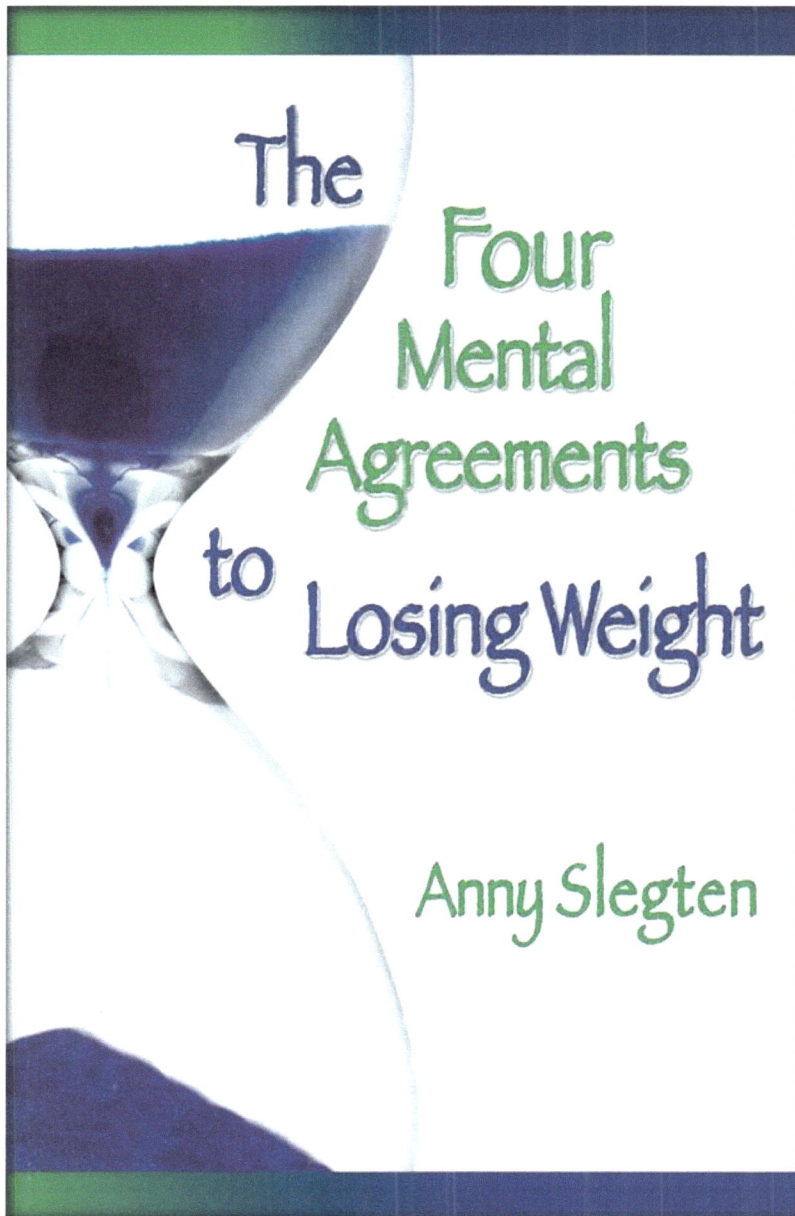

The Four Mental Agreements
To Losing Weight
http://www.connectwithanny.com

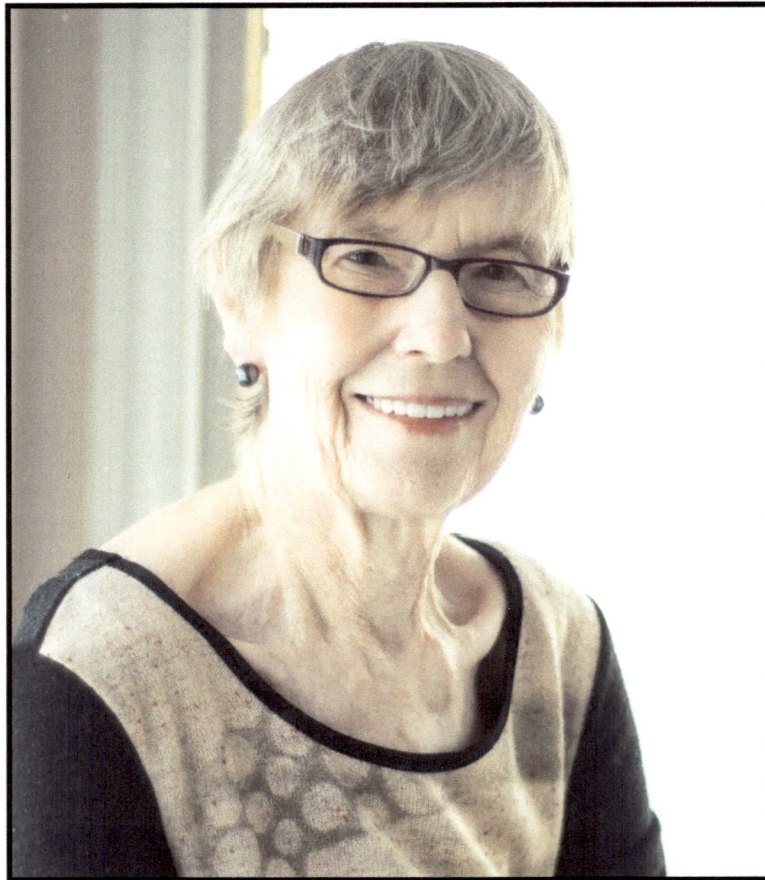

About The Author

As Director of The Hypnotism Training Institute of Alberta and The Reiki Training Centre of Canada, Anny has developed and structured the training and curriculum to the highest standards for both The Hypnotism Training Institute of Alberta and the Reiki Training Centre of Canada. She offers training to students that come from all over Canada and around the world.

Anny has experienced and lived in many corners of the globe and this has given her a unique understanding of many cultures.

Anny's Belgian parents were from the Flemish part of Belgium and were speaking Flemish (Dutch) at home. Living in Congo, everything was in French.

Although she never spoke Flemish (Dutch), Anny speaks English with a guttural Dutch/German accent. Living in the English-speaking part of Canada for decades, Anny now speaks French with an English accent!

Anny is an Author and holds certifications as:

Master Hypnotist
Clinical Hypnotherapist
Hypno-Baby Birthing Facilitator and Instructor
HypnoBirthing™ Fertility Therapist for Men & Women
Reiki Master/Teacher
Master Remote Viewer

Anny is a world renowned Clinical Hypnotherapist and Hypnologist in full time practice since 1984 as well as a Hypno-Energy worker since 2008.

In 1986 Anny created and developed an unique method using hypnosis for distance services - Virtual Sessions.

Over the years these Virtual Sessions proved to be an effective, useful, and efficient method for investigations and putting closure on both present and past issues - resulting in peace of mind.

To know more about Anny, please visit www.annyslegten.com and make sure to read what she published on her Blog.

Do you wonder what else Anny is publishing?

Visit http://www.connectwithanny.com

www.success-and-more.com

www.ingramcontent.com/pod-product-compliance
Lightning Source LLC
Chambersburg PA
CBHW050814220326
41598CB00006B/203